C000187001

Delicious Comfort Food for People In a Hurry

Fit and healthy comfort food recipes for each time of the day

Andrew Tyle

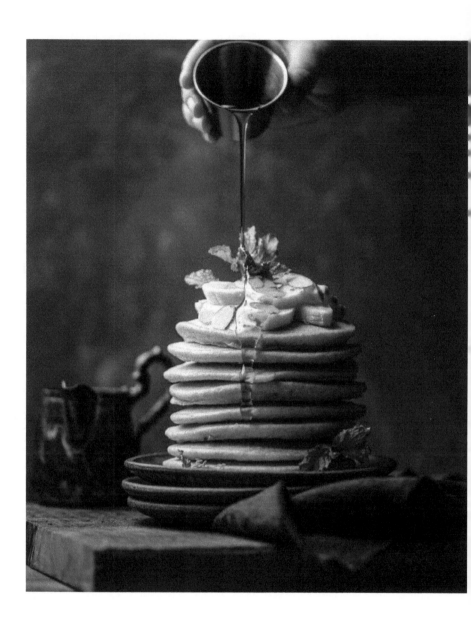

professional advice. The content within this book has been derived from various sources. Please consult a licensed professional before attempting any techniques outlined in this book.

By reading this document, the reader agrees that under no circumstances is the author responsible for any losses, direct or indirect, which are incurred as a result of the use of information contained within this document, including, but not limited to, — errors, omissions, or inaccuracies.

Table of Contents

Mini Veggie Quiche

Preparation Time: 10 minutes | Cooking Time: 20 minutes | Servings: 12

Ingredients:

6 eggs

1/4 cup bell pepper, diced

3/4 cup cheddar cheese, shredded

10 oz frozen spinach, chopped

1/4 cup onion, chopped

1/4 cup mushroom, diced

Directions:

Add all ingredients into the large bowl and whisk until combined.

Pour egg mixture into the 12 silicone muffin molds.

Place the dehydrating tray in a multi-level air fryer basket and place basket in the Pressure Pot.

Place 6 muffin molds on a dehydrating tray.

Seal pot with air fryer lid and select bake mode then set the temperature to 350 F and timer for 20 minutes.

Bake remaining muffins using the same method.

Serve and enjoy.

Nutrition:

Calories 67, Fat 4.6 g, Carbohydrates 1.6 g, Sugar 0.6 g, Protein 5.3 g, Cholesterol 89 mg

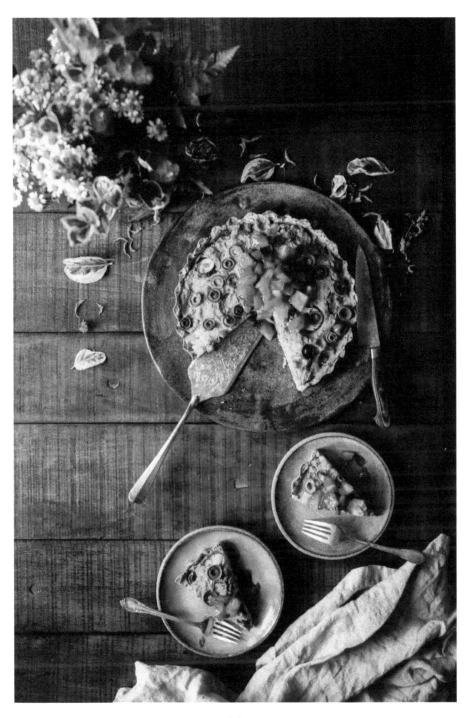

Broccoli Cheese Loaf

Preparation Time: 10 minutes | Cooking Time: 30 minutes | Servings: 4

Ingredients:

5 eggs, lightly beaten

3/4 cup broccoli florets, chopped

1 cup cheddar cheese, shredded

2 tsp baking powder

3 1/1 tbsp coconut flour

1 tsp salt

Directions:

Spray a loaf pan with cooking spray and set aside.

Add all ingredients into the bowl and mix well.

Pour egg mixture into the prepared loaf pan.

Place steam rack into the Pressure Pot then places loaf pan on top of the rack.

Seal pot with air fryer lid and select bake mode then set the temperature to 350 F and timer for 30 minutes.

Serve and enjoy.

Nutrition:

Calories 231, Fat 15.7 g, Carbohydrates 8.1 g, Sugar 0.9 g, Protein 15.4 g, Cholesterol 234 mg

Chicken Casserole

Preparation Time: 10 minutes | Cooking Time: 25 minutes | Servings: 8

Ingredients:

2 lbs cooked chicken, shredded

6 oz cream cheese, softened

4 oz butter, melted

6 oz ham, cut into small pieces

5 oz Swiss cheese

1 oz fresh lemon juice

1 tbsp Dijon mustard

1/2 tsp salt

Directions:

Spray Pressure Pot from inside with cooking spray.

Add chicken and ham into the Pressure Pot and spread evenly.

Add butter, lemon juice, mustard, cream cheese, and salt into the blender and blend until a thick sauce.

Spread sauce over top of chicken and ham mixture.

Arrange Swiss cheese slices on top of the sauce.

Seal pot with air fryer lid and select bake mode then set the temperature to 350 F and timer for 25 minutes.

Serve and enjoy.

Nutrition:

Calories 451, Fat 29.2 g, Carbohydrates 2.5 g, Sugar 0.4 g, Protein 43g, Cholesterol 170 mg.

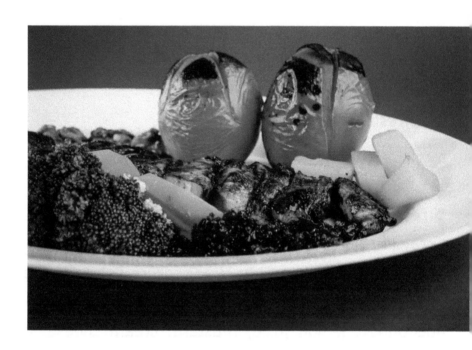

Baked Chicken & Mushrooms

Preparation Time: 10 minutes | Cooking Time: 30 minutes | Servings: 2

Ingredients:

2 chicken breasts, boneless and skinless

1/4 cup sun-dried tomatoes

4 oz mushrooms, sliced

1/4 cup mayonnaise

1/2 tsp salt

Directions:

Line Pressure Pot multi-level air fryer basket with foil.

Brush chicken breast with mayonnaise and place it into the air fryer basket and place the basket into the Pressure Pot.

Add sun-dried tomatoes, mushrooms, and salt on top of the chicken.

Seal pot with air fryer lid and select bake mode then set the temperature to 380 F and timer for 30 minutes.

Serve and enjoy.

Nutrition:

Calories 408, Fat 20.8 g, Carbohydrates 9.8 g, Sugar 3.4 g, Protein 44.5 g, Cholesterol 138 mg.

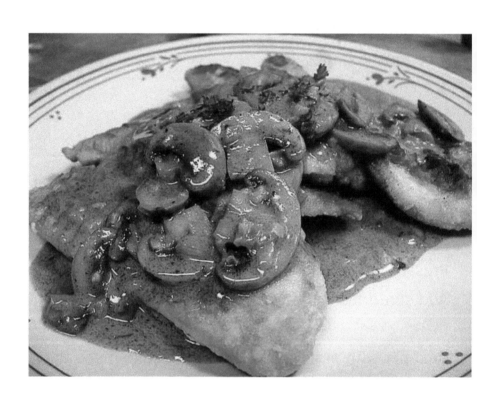

Bacon Egg Muffins

Preparation Time: 10 minutes | Cooking Time: 25 minutes | Servings: 12

Ingredients:

12 eggs

8 bacon slices, cooked and crumbled

2 tbsp fresh parsley, chopped

1/2 tsp mustard powder

1/3 cup heavy cream

2 green onion, chopped

4 oz cheddar cheese, shredded

Pepper

Salt

Directions:

In a mixing bowl, whisk together eggs, mustard powder, heavy cream, pepper, and salt.

Divide cheddar cheese, onions, and bacon into the 12 silicone muffin molds.

Pour egg mixture into the muffin molds.

Place the dehydrating tray in a multi-level air fryer basket and place basket in the Pressure Pot.

Place 6 muffin molds on a dehydrating tray.

Seal pot with air fryer lid and select bake mode then set the temperature to 375 F and timer for 25 minutes.

Serve and enjoy.

Nutrition:

Calories 183, Fat 14.1 g, Carbohydrates 1 g, Sugar 0.5 g, Protein 12.8 g, Cholesterol 192 mg.

Sweet Squash Breakfast

Preparation time: 10 minutes | Cooking Time: 4 minutes | Servings: 4

Ingredients:

1 ½ cups coconut milk, unsweetened

A pinch of ground cloves

A pinch of ground nutmeg

1 small zucchini, grated

5 oz squash, grated

2 tablespoons swerve

½ teaspoon ground cinnamon

¼ cup chopped pecans

Directions:

In your Pressure Pot, mix milk with cloves, nutmeg, zucchini, squash, swerve, cinnamon and pecans. Stir, cover, and cook on High pressure for 4 minutes.

Divide into bowls and serve hot.

Enjoy!

Nutrition:

Calories 100, fat 1g, fiber 2g, carbs 3g, Protein 4g.

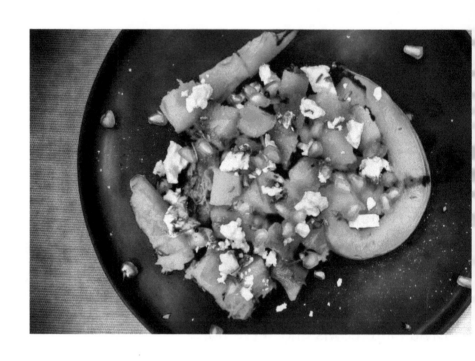

Okra and Zucchini Breakfast

Preparation time: 10 minutes | Cooking Time: 10 minutes | Servings: 4

Ingredients:

1 ½ cups chopped red onion

3 tablespoons olive oil

2 cups sliced okra

1 cup sliced mushrooms

1 cup cherry tomatoes, halved

1 cup of water

2 cups chopped zucchini

2 cups chopped yellow bell pepper

Black pepper to the taste

2 tablespoons chopped basil

1 tablespoon chopped thyme

½ cup balsamic vinegar

Directions:

Put onion, tomato, okra, mushrooms, zucchini, bell pepper, basil, thyme, vinegar, and oil in your Pressure Pot and toss.

Add black pepper, toss again then add the water. Cover pot and cook on High pressure for 10 minutes.

Divide between plates and serve for breakfast.

Enjoy!

Nutrition:

Calories 120, fat 2g, fiber 2g, carbs 3g, Protein 6g.

Pumpkin Oatmeal

Preparation Time: 10 minutes | Cooking Time: 10 minutes | Servings: 4

Ingredients:

1 cup steel-cut oats

2 tbsp maple syrup

1/4 cup pumpkin

1/4 tsp cinnamon

1 tbsp brown sugar

1 tsp vanilla

1 1/4 cups water

14 oz can coconut milk

1/2 tsp salt

Directions:

Add oats, vanilla, water, coconut milk, and salt into the Pressure Pot and stir well.

Seal pot with the lid and select manual high pressure for 10 minutes.

Release pressure using the quick-release method than open the lid.

Stir in cinnamon, brown sugar, maple syrup, and pumpkin.

Serve and enjoy.

Nutrition:

Calorie 187, Carbohydrates 25.9g, Protein 4.5g, Fat 7.2g, Sugar 10.6g, Sodium 303mg.

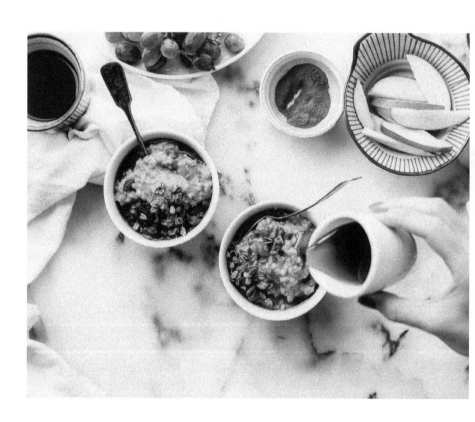

Pressure Pot Eggs in Marinara Sauce

Preparation Time: 5 minutes | Cooking Time: 10 minutes | Servings: 2

Ingredients:

1 tablespoon coconut oil

2 cloves of garlic, minced

½ onion, diced

1 red bell pepper, diced

1 teaspoon chili powder

½ teaspoon paprika

½ teaspoon ground cumin

Salt and pepper to taste

1 ½ cups commercial marinara sauce

6 eggs

Parsley leaves for garnish

Directions:

Press the Sauté button on the Pressure Pot.

Sauté the garlic and onions until fragrant.

Add the bell pepper, chili powder, paprika, and cumin.

Season with salt and pepper to taste.

Continue stirring for 3 minutes.

Pour in the marinara sauce.

Gently crack the eggs into the marinara sauce.

Close the lid.

Press the Manual button and adjust the cooking time to 10 minutes.

Do natural pressure release.

1Once the lid is opened, garnish with parsley.

Nutrition:

Calories 182, Carbohydrates 8.4 g, Protein 10.6g, Fat 12.2g, Fiber 1.8g.

Indian Scrambled Eggs

Preparation Time: 5 minutes | Cooking Time:3 minutes | Servings: 4

Ingredients:

6 eggs

¼ cup milk

1 tablespoon cooking oil

1 tablespoon ghee

1 large onion, chopped

2 cloves of garlic, minced

1 tomato, chopped

1 jalapeno pepper, chopped

½ inch ginger, grated

3 scallions, chopped

¼ teaspoon ground turmeric

1 teaspoon garam masala

Directions:

In a mixing bowl, combine the eggs and milk. Set aside.

Press the Sauté button on the Pressure Pot.

Heat the oil and ghee.

Sauté the onion and garlic until fragrant.

Add the tomatoes, pepper, ginger, scallions, turmeric, and garam masala. Continue stirring for 3 minutes.

27

Add the egg mixture.

Give a good stir.

Close the lid.

Press the Manual button and adjust the cooking time to 3 minutes.

Do natural pressure release.

Once the lid is open, fluff the eggs using two forks.

Nutrition:

Calories 162, Carbohydrates 8.3g, Protein 9.7g, Fat 10.3g. Fiber 4.2g.

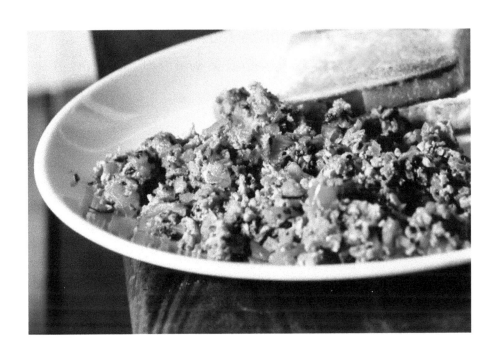

Eggs and Chorizo

Preparation Time: 5 minutes | Cooking Time: 10 minutes | Servings: 4

Ingredients:

1 tablespoon olive oil

1/3 cup onions, chopped

¼ pounds Mexican chorizo sausage, chopped

3 tablespoon raisins, soaked in water then drained

6 eggs

Salt and pepper to taste

Directions:

Press the Sauté button on the Pressure Pot.

Heat the oil and sauté the onions until fragrant.

Add in the chorizo sausages and continue stirring for 3 minutes.

Stir in the raisins and eggs

Season with salt and pepper to taste.

Close the lid and press the Manual button.

Adjust the cooking time to 10 minutes.

Do natural pressure release.

Nutrition:

Calories 409, Carbohydrates 8.8g, Protein 25.4g, Fat 30.7g, Fiber 1.5g.

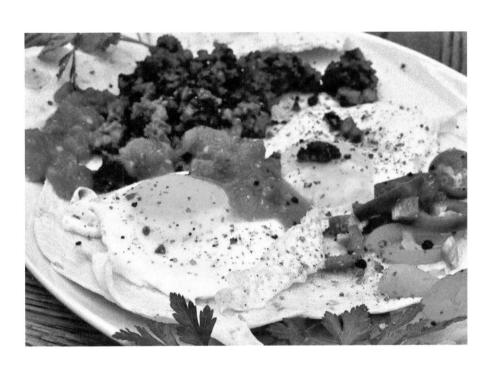

Asian Scrambled Eggs

Preparation Time: 5 minutes | Cooking Time: 15 minutes | Servings: 4

Ingredients:

4 large eggs, beaten

1 tablespoon light soy sauce

½ teaspoon oyster sauce

2 tomatoes, sliced

1 tablespoon oil

½ cup chicken stock

1 tablespoon potato starch

Directions:

In a mixing bowl, mix all ingredients until well combined.

Pour over the Pressure Pot.

Close the lid and press the Manual button.

Adjust the cooking time to 15 minutes.

Do natural pressure release.

Once the lid is open, fluff the eggs using a fork.

Nutrition:

Calories 278, Carbohydrates 13.4g, Protein 15.6g, Fat 17.2g, Fiber 1.8g.

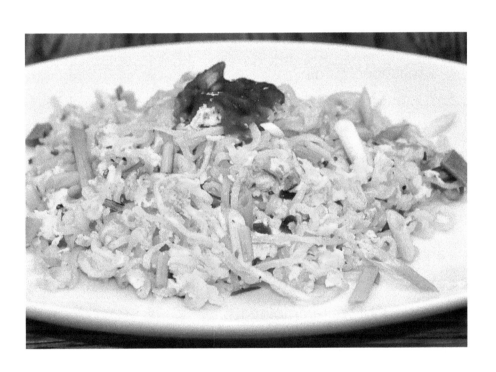

Pressure Pot Poblano Cheese Frittata

Preparation Time: 5 minutes | Cooking Time: 10 minutes | Servings: 4

Ingredients:

4 eggs

1 cup half and half

½ teaspoon salt

½ teaspoon cumin

10 ounces canned green chilies, chopped

1 cup Mexican cheese blend, grated

½ cup cilantro, chopped

Directions:

Place a trivet or steamer basket inside the Pressure Pot and pour water over. In a mixing bowl, combine the eggs and half-and-half. Season with salt and cumin. Whisk until well-combined.

Place the egg mixture into a baking dish that will fit inside the Pressure Pot.

Add the chilies and top with a Mexican cheese blend.

Cover the baking dish with aluminum foil.

Place the baking dish with the egg mixture on the steamer basket.

Close the lid.

Press the Manual button and adjust the cooking time to 10 minutes.

Do natural pressure release.

Garnish with chopped cilantro.

Nutrition:

Calories 257, Carbohydrates 6g, Protein 14.2g, Fat 19g, Fiber 1.5g.

Herbed Crustless Quiche

Preparation Time: 5 minutes | Cooking Time: 15 minutes | Servings: 8

Ingredients:

4 eggs

1 cup milk

1/3 cup flour

¼ teaspoon baking soda

½ teaspoon salt

½ teaspoon thyme

1 tablespoon parsley

1/8 teaspoon paprika

A dash of crushed red pepper

½ teaspoon dill

Salt and pepper to taste

1 cup spinach, chopped

2 scallions, chopped

½ cup broccoli, chopped

½ red bell pepper, chopped

½ cup goat cheese, cubed

Directions:

Place a trivet or steamer basket inside the Pressure Pot and pour water over.

In a mixing bowl, combine the eggs, milk, flour, baking soda, salt, thyme, parsley, paprika, crushed red pepper, and dill. Season with salt and pepper to taste.

Place the egg mixture into a baking dish that will fit inside the Pressure Pot.

Stir in the spinach, scallions, broccoli, red bell pepper, and goat cheese.

Cover the baking dish with aluminum foil.

Place the baking dish with the egg mixture on the steamer basket.

Close the lid.

Press the Manual button and adjust the cooking time to 15 minutes.

Do natural pressure release.

Nutrition:

Calories 122, Carbohydrates 7.9g, Protein 7.3g, Fat 6.8g, Fiber 0.7g.

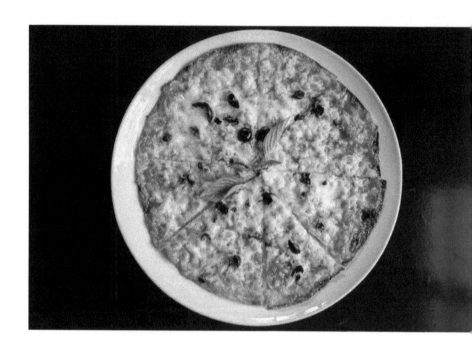

Lemony Raspberries Bowls

Preparation time: 17 minutes | Cooking Time: 15 minutes | Servings: 2

Ingredients:

1 cup raspberries

2 tbsp. Butter

2 tbsp. Lemon juice

1 tsp. Cinnamon powder

Directions:

In your air fryer, mix all the ingredients, toss, cover, cook at 350°f for 12 minutes.

Divide into bowls and serve for breakfast.

Nutrition:

Calories 208, Fat 6g, Fiber 9g, Carbs 14g, Protein 3g.

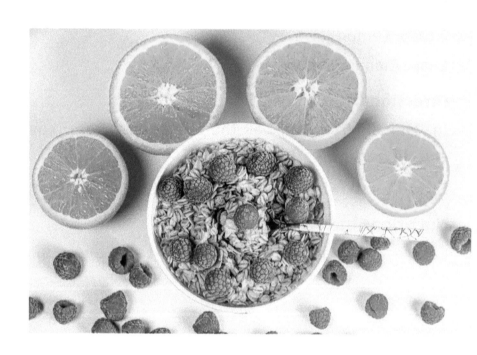

Spaghetti Squash Fritters

Preparation time: 23 minutes | Cooking Time: 15 minutes | Servings: 4

Ingredients:

2 cups cooked spaghetti squash

2 stalks green onion, sliced

1 large egg.

¼ cup blanched finely ground almond flour.

2 tbsp. Unsalted butter; softened.

½ tsp. Garlic powder.

1 tsp. Dried parsley.

Directions:

Remove excess moisture from the squash using a cheesecloth or kitchen towel.

Mix all ingredients in a large bowl. Form into four patties.

Cut a piece of parchment to fit your air fryer basket. Place each patty on the parchment and place it into the air fryer basket.

Adjust the temperature to 400° F and set the timer for 8 minutes.

Flip the patties halfway through the cooking time.

Serve warm.

Nutrition:

Calories 131, Protein 3.8g, Fiber 2.0g, Fat 10.1g, Carbs 7.1g.

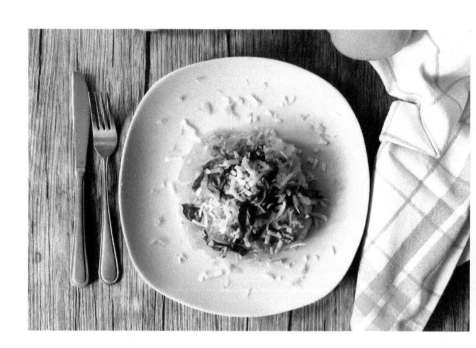

Zucchini Fritters

Preparation time: 13 minutes | Cooking Time: 15 minutes | Servings: 4

Ingredients:

2 eggs; whisked

8 oz. Zucchinis; chopped.

2 spring onions; chopped.

¼ tsp. Sweet paprika; chopped.

Cooking spray

Salt and black pepper to taste.

Directions:

Take a bowl and mix all the ingredients except the cooking spray, stir well and shape medium fritters out of this mix.

Put the basket in the air fryer, add the fritters inside, grease them with cooking spray, and cook at 400°f for 8 minutes.

Divide the fritters between plates and serve for breakfast.

Nutrition:

Calories 202, Fat 10g, Fiber 2g, Carbs 4g, Protein 5g.

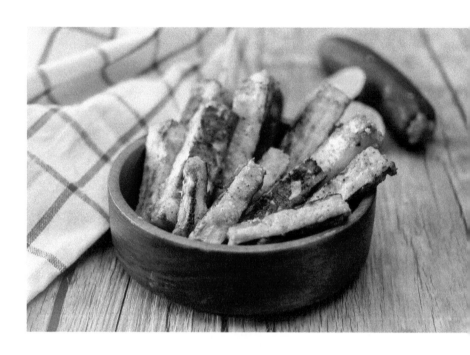

Ground Pork with Eggs Frittata

Preparation Time: 7Minutes | Cooking Time:13Minutes | Servings: 4

Ingredients:

2 tbsp ghee

1 onion, finely chopped

1 lb ground pork grass-fed

6 free-range eggs

2 Tbsp fresh cilantro, roughly chopped

Salt and ground black pepper to taste

1 cup water for Pressure Pot

Directions

Press the SAUTÉ button on your Pressure Pot.

When the word "hot" appears on the display, heat ghee and sauté the onions for about 3 - 4 minutes.

Add the ground pork and sauté with a pinch of salt for 2 minutes.

Sprinkle fresh cilantro, stir and press the Stop button.

Whisk the eggs in a bowl with a pinch of salt and pepper.

Pour eggs in your Pressure Pot and stir.

Lock lid into place and set on the MANUAL setting for 5 minutes.

Use Quick Release - turn the valve from sealing to venting to release the pressure.

Serve hot.

Nutrition:

Calories 253, Fat 11.o3g, Carbohydrates 0.93g, Fiber 0.17g, Protein 34.95g.

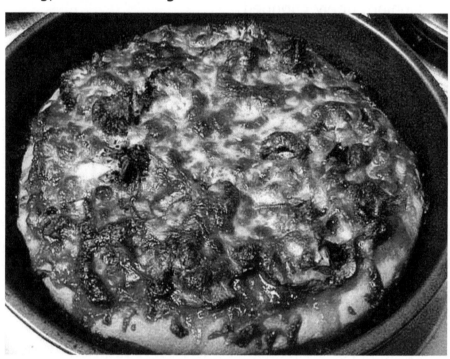

Italian Turkey Sausage Muffins

Preparation Time: 5Minutes | Cooking Time:15Minutes | Servings: 4

Ingredients:

1 lb Turkey Italian sausage

2 cups chopped kale

6 pastured eggs

1/4 cup Extra Virgin Olive oil

2 cloves garlic

2 Tbsp Italian seasoning

2 Tbsp dried minced onion

Sea salt and ground black pepper to taste

1 cup water for Pressure Pot

Directions:

Place the kale leaves, eggs, olive oil, garlic, Italian seasoning, onion, salt, and pepper in your blender and pulse/ blend for about 1 minute, or until thoroughly mixed.

Transfer to a large bowl and stir in the sausage until well mixed.

Fill the muffin tins to just beneath the rim.

Pour water into the inner stainless-steel pot in the Pressure Pot, and place the trivets inside a steam rack or a steamer basket.

Place muffin tins on a trivet.

Lock lid into place and set on the MANUAL setting for 10 minutes.

When the beep sounds, quick release the pressure by pressing Cancel, and twisting the steam handle to the Venting position.

Serve hot or cold.

Nutrition:

Calories 349.23, Fat 28.77g, Carbohydrates 5.27g, Fiber 0.72g, Protein 18.61g.

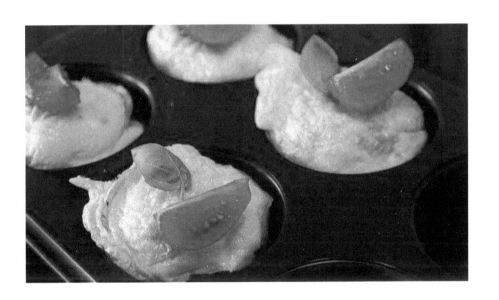

Mustard Eggs and Avocado Mash

Preparation Time: 5Minutes | Cooking Time: 10Minutes | Servings: 4

Ingredients:

2 cups water for Pressure Pot

6 free-range eggs

1/2 cup stone-ground mustard

1 avocado, chopped

1 tsp of lemon juice, freshly squeezed

1 Tbsp fresh chopped parsley optional

Salt and pepper, to taste

Directions:

Pour water into the inner stainless-steel pot in the Pressure Pot and place the steamer basket.

Lock lid into place and set on the MANUAL setting for 5 minutes.

It will take the cooker approximately 5 minutes to build to pressure and then 5 minutes to cook.

Use Quick Release - turn the valve from sealing to venting to release the pressure.

Place the eggs in cold water and peel. Cut the eggs into small pieces and season with salt and pepper.

Wash, peel, and clean avocado.

Mash avocado with the fork, and sprinkle with salt and pepper.

Combine the eggs, mustard, mashed avocado, lemon juice, and fresh parsley.

Refrigerate for one hour and serve.

Nutrition:

Calories 161, Fat 12.05g, Carbohydrates 4.97g, Fiber: 3.24g, Protein 9.35g.

Apple Cinnamon Oatmeal

Preparation Time: 10 minutes | Cooking Time: 4 minutes | Servings: 4

Ingredients:

2 cups steel-cut oats

1/4 tsp nutmeg

1 1/2 tsp cinnamon

2 apples, diced

4 1/2 cups water

Directions:

Add all ingredients into the Pressure Pot and stir well.

Seal pot with lid and cook on manual high pressure for 4 minutes.

Once done then allow to release pressure naturally for 10 minutes then release using the quick-release method. Open the lid.

Stir well and serve.

Nutrition:

Calories 216, Fat 2.9 g, Carbohydrates 43.9 g, Sugar 12.1 g, Protein 5.7 g, Cholesterol 0 mg.

Roasted Potatoes

Preparation Time: 5Minutes | Cooking Time: 12 Minutes | Servings: 4

Ingredients:

1 1/2 lbs russet potatoes, cut into wedges

1 cup chicken stock

1/2 tsp onion powder

4 tbsp olive oil

1/4 tsp paprika

1 tsp garlic powder

1/4 tsp pepper

1 tsp sea salt

Directions:

Add oil in the Pressure Pot and select sauté.

Add potatoes in the pot and sauté for 5-6 minutes.

Add remaining ingredients into the pot and stir well.

Seal pot with lid and cook on high pressure for 6 minutes.

Release pressure using the quick-release method then open the lid carefully.

Stir well and serve.

Nutrition:

Calories 244, Carbohydrates 27.8g, Protein 3.2g, Fat, 14.3g, Sugar 2.4g, Sodium 670mg.

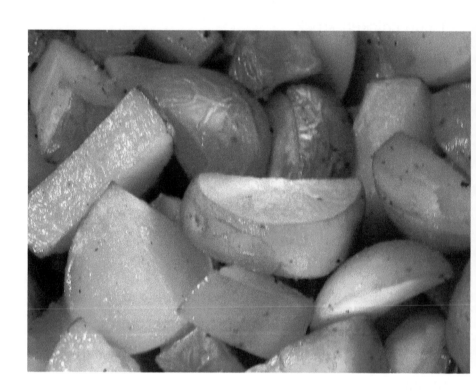

Brussels sprouts with Nut

Preparation Time: 5 Minutes | Cooking Time: 3 Minutes | Servings: 4

Ingredients:

1 lb Brussels sprouts

4 tbsp pine nuts

1 cup of water

1/2 tbsp olive oil

Pepper

Salt

Directions:

Pour water into the Pressure Pot.

Add Brussels sprouts to a steamer basket and place the basket in the pot.

Seal pot with lid and cook on manual high pressure for 3 minutes.

Release pressure using the quick-release method. Open the lid carefully.

Season with pepper and salt. Drizzle with olive oil.

Sprinkle pine nuts and serve.

Nutrition:

Calories 122, Carbohydrates 11.5g, Protein 5.1g, Fat 8g, Sugar 2.8g, Sodium 69mg.

Classic Frittata

Preparation time: 10 minutes | Cooking Time: 5 minutes | Servings: 6

Ingredients:

2 tablespoons almond milk

A pinch of black pepper

6 eggs, whisked

2 tablespoons parsley, chopped

1 tablespoon low-fat cheese, shredded

Cooking spray

1 cup of water

Directions:

In a bowl, mix the eggs with the almond milk, black pepper, parsley, and cheese and whisk well.

Grease a pan that fits your Pressure Pot with cooking spray and pour the egg mix into the pan.

Add the water to your Pressure Pot, add the steamer basket, add the pan inside, cover, and cook on High for 5 minutes.

Divide the frittata between plates and serve.

Enjoy!

Nutrition:

Calories 200, fat 4g, fiber 6g, carb 17g, Protein 6g.

Simple Baked Eggs

Preparation time: 10 minutes | Cooking Time: 4 minutes | Servings: 4

Ingredients:

4 eggs

4 slices of low-fat cheddar

2 spring onions, chopped

1 tablespoon olive oil

1 tablespoon cilantro, chopped

1 cup of water

Directions:

Grease 4 ramekins with the oil, sprinkle green onions in each, crack an egg in each ramekin, and top with cilantro and cheddar cheese.

Add the water to your Pressure Pot, add steamer basket, add the ramekins inside, cover, and cook on Low for 4 minutes.

Serve the eggs right away for breakfast.

Enjoy!

Nutrition:

Calories 211, fat 3g, fiber 7g, carbs 18g, Protein 5g.

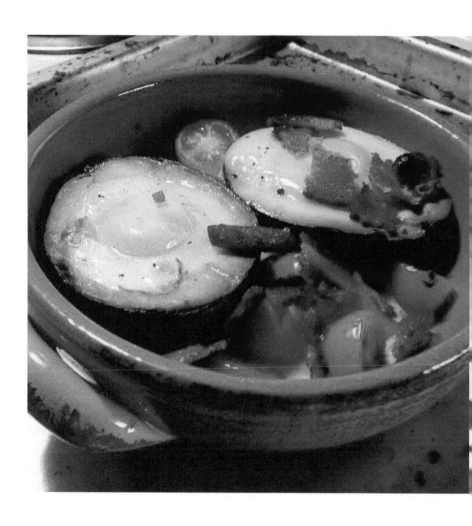

Mexican Casserole

Preparation time: 10 minutes | Cooking Time: 20 minutes | Servings: 8

Ingredients:

8 eggs, whisked

2 red onion, chopped

1 pound chicken sausage, chopped

1 red bell pepper, chopped

4 ounces canned black beans, no-salt-added, drained and rinsed

½ cup green onions, chopped

½ cup whole wheat flour

1 cup low-fat mozzarella cheese, shredded

Directions:

Set your Pressure Pot on sauté mode, add onion and sausage, stir and brown for 4-5 minutes.

Add eggs, flour, red bell pepper, beans, green onions, and stir.

Sprinkle the mozzarella all over, cover the pot and cook on High for 20 minutes.

Divide the mix between plates and serve for breakfast. Enjoy!

Nutrition:

Calories 199, fat 3g, fiber 6g, carbs 17g, Protein 8g.

Poached Eggs

Preparation time: 10 minutes | Cooking Time: 4 minutes | Servings: 2

Ingredients:

2 slices of low-fat mozzarella

2 eggs

1 bell pepper, tops cut off and halved

2/3 cup mayonnaise

3 tablespoons orange juice

1 and ½ teaspoons mustard

1 teaspoon lemon juice

1 tablespoon vinegar

1 teaspoon turmeric powder

1 cup of water

Directions:

Crack the eggs in bell pepper cups and top each with a mozzarella slice.

Add the water to your Pressure Pot, add steamer basket, add bell pepper cups, cover, and cook on Low for 4 minutes.

In a bowl, mix the mayonnaise with the orange juice, mustard, lemon juice, vinegar, and turmeric and whisk well.

Divide the poached eggs between plates, spread the sauce you've made all over, and serve.

Enjoy!

Nutrition:

Calories 199, fat 3g, fiber 5g, carbs 20g, Protein 4g.

Eggs and Hash Browns

Preparation time: 10 minutes | Cooking Time: 20 minutes | Servings: 6

Ingredients:

1 cup of water

Cooking spray

6 eggs

2 cups hash browns

¼ cup almond milk

½ cup fat-free cheddar cheese, shredded

1 small yellow onion, chopped

A pinch of black pepper

½ green bell pepper, chopped

½ red bell pepper, chopped

Directions:

Grease a pan that fits your Pressure Pot with cooking spray, add hash browns, onion, black pepper, red bell pepper, and green bell pepper, and toss.

In a bowl, mix the eggs with cheese and milk and whisk well.

Pour this into the pan and toss gently.

Add the water to your Pressure Pot, add steamer basket, add the pan inside, cover, and cook on High for 20 minutes.

Divide the mix between plates and serve.

Enjoy!

Nutrition:

Calories 221, fat 4g, fiber 5g, carbs 22g, Protein 6g.

Delicious Egg Risotto

Preparation time: 10 minutes | Cooking Time: 12 minutes | Servings: 2

Ingredients:

3 slices bacon, low-sodium, and chopped

1 cup white rice

1/3 cup yellow onion, chopped

1 and ½ cups low-sodium chicken stock

2 eggs, fried

2 tablespoons low-fat parmesan, grated

1 tablespoon chives, chopped

A pinch of black pepper

Directions:

Set your Pressure Pot on sauté mode, add bacon, stir and cook for 2-3 minutes.

Add the onion, stir and cook for 2 minutes more.

Add rice, stock, black pepper, and parmesan, cover, and cook on High for 7 minutes more.

Divide the risotto between plates, top with the eggs, sprinkle chives on top, and serve for breakfast.

Enjoy!

Nutrition:

Calories 212, fat 5g, fiber 8g, carbs 19g, Protein 6g.

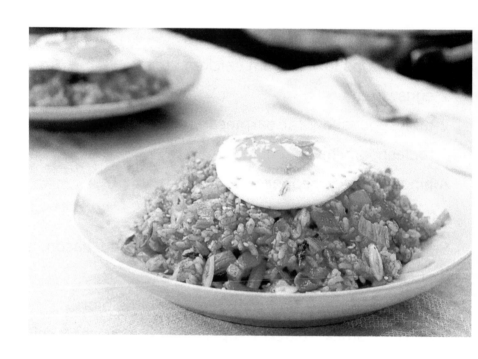

Creamy Cauliflower Mashed

Preparation Time: 10 minutes | Cooking Time: 15 minutes | Servings: 4

Ingredients:

1 medium cauliflower head, cut into florets

2 tbsp heavy cream

1/4 tsp garlic powder

1/4 tsp onion powder

4 tbsp butter

1 1/2 tbsp ranch seasoning

1 cup of water

Directions:

Pour water into the Pressure Pot.

Add cauliflower florets into the steamer basket and place the basket in the pot.

Seal the pot with a pressure-cooking lid and cook on high for 15 minutes.

Once done, release pressure using a quick release. Remove lid.

Transfer cauliflower florets into the mixing bowl.

Add remaining ingredients and mash cauliflower mixture until smooth.

Serve and enjoy.

Nutrition:

Calories 176, Fat 14.4 g, Carbohydrates 8.1 g, Sugar 3.6 g, Protein 3.2 g, Cholesterol 41 mg.

Spicy Cabbage

Preparation Time: 10 minutes | Cooking Time: 5 minutes | Servings: 6

Ingredients:

1 cabbage head, chopped

2 tbsp olive oil

1 tsp chili powder

3 tbsp soy sauce

1/2 onion, diced

1 tsp paprika

1/2 tsp garlic salt

1 cup vegetable stock

1/2 tsp salt

Directions:

Add oil into the inner pot of Pressure Pot duo crisp and set pot on sauté mode.

Add cabbage and sauté for 1-2 minutes.

Add remaining ingredients and stir everything well.

Seal the pot with a pressure-cooking lid and cook on high for 3 minutes.

Once done, release pressure using a quick release. Remove lid.

Stir and serve.

Nutrition:

Calories 82, Fat 4.9 g, Carbohydrates 9.1 g, Sugar 4.6 g, Protein 2.3 g, Cholesterol 0 mg

Salmon Quiche

Preparation time: 15 minutes | Cooking Time: 20 minutes | Servings: 2

Ingredients:

5½ oz. Salmon fillet, chopped

Salt and ground black pepper, as required

½ tablespoon fresh lemon juice

1 egg yolk

3½ tablespoons chilled butter

2/3 cup flour

1 tablespoon cold water

2 eggs

3 tablespoons whipping cream

1 scallion, chopped

Directions:

In a bowl, mix the salmon, salt, black pepper, and lemon juice.

In another bowl, add the egg yolk, butter, flour, and water and mix until a dough form.

Place the dough onto a floured smooth surface and roll into about a 7-inch round.

Place the dough in a quiche pan and press firmly in the bottom and along the edges.

Trim the excess edges.

In a small bowl, add the eggs, cream, salt, and black pepper and beat until well combined.

Place the cream mixture over the crust evenly and top with the salmon mixture, followed by the scallion.

Press the "power button" of the air fry oven and turn the dial to select the "air fry" mode.

Press the time button and again turn the dial to set the cooking time to 20 minutes.

Now push the temp button and rotate the dial to set the temperature at 355 degrees f.

Press the "start/pause" button to start.

When the unit beeps to show that it is preheated, open the lid.

Arrange pan over the "wire rack" and insert in the oven. Cut into equal-sized wedges and serve.

Nutrition:

Calories 592, Total fat 39g, Saturated fat 20.1g, Cholesterol 381mg, Sodium 331mg, Total carbs 33.8g, Fiber 1.4g, Sugar 0.8g, Protein 27.2g.

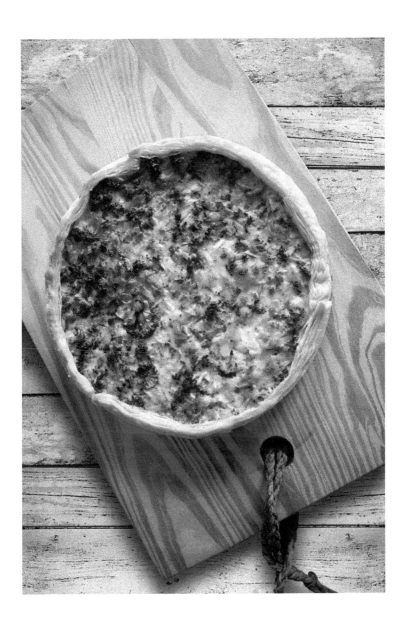

Bacon & Spinach Quiche

Preparation time: 15 minutes | Cooking Time: 10 minutes | Servings: 4

Ingredients:

2 cooked bacon slices, chopped

½ cup fresh spinach, chopped

¼ cup mozzarella cheese, shredded

½ cup parmesan cheese, shredded

2 tablespoons milk

2 dashes of tabasco sauce

Salt and ground black pepper, as required

Directions:

In a bowl, add all ingredients and mix well.

Transfer the mixture into a baking pan.

Press the "power button" of the air fry oven and turn the dial to select the "air fry" mode.

Press the time button and again turn the dial to set the cooking time to 10 minutes.

Now push the temp button and rotate the dial to set the temperature at 320° F.

Press the "start/pause" button to start.

When the unit beeps to show that it is preheated, open the lid.

Arrange pan over the "wire rack" and insert in the oven. Cut into equal-sized wedges and serve hot.

Nutrition:

Calories 130, Total fat 9.3g, Saturated fat 4g, Cholesterol 25mg, Sodium 561mg, Total carbs 1.1g, Fiber 0.1g, Sugar 0.4g, Protein 10g.

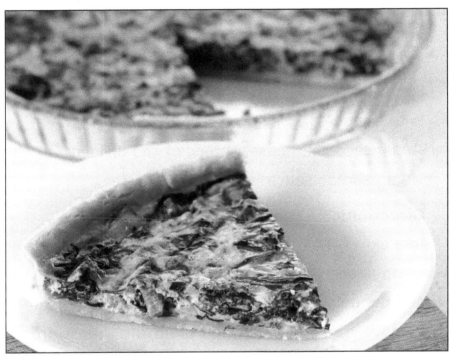

Sausage & Mushroom Casserole

Preparation time: 15 minutes | Cooking Time: 19 minutes | Servings: 6

Ingredients:

1 tablespoon olive oil

½ lb. Spicy ground sausage

¾ cup yellow onion, chopped

5 fresh mushrooms, sliced

8 eggs, beaten

½ teaspoon garlic salt

¾ cup cheddar cheese, shredded and divided

¼ cup alfredo sauce

Directions:

In a skillet, heat the oil over medium heat and cook the sausage and onions for about 4-5 minutes.

Add the mushrooms and cook for about 6-7 minutes.

Remove from the oven and drain the grease from the skillet.

In a bowl, add the sausage mixture, beaten eggs, garlic salt, ½ cup of cheese, and alfredo sauce and stir to combine.

Place the sausage mixture into a baking pan.

Press the "power button" of the air fry oven and turn the dial to select the "air fry" mode.

Press the time button and again turn the dial to set the cooking time to 12 minutes.

Now push the temp button and rotate the dial to set the temperature at 390° F.

Press the "start/pause" button to start.

When the unit beeps to show that it is preheated, open the lid.

Arrange pan over the "wire rack" and insert in the oven.

After 6 minutes of cooking, stir the sausage mixture well.

Cut into equal-sized wedges and serve with the topping of remaining cheese.

Nutrition:

Calories 319, Total fat 24.5g, Saturated fat 9.1g, Cholesterol 267mg, Sodium 698mg, Total carbs 5g, Fiber 0.5g, Sugar 1.5g, Protein 19.7g.

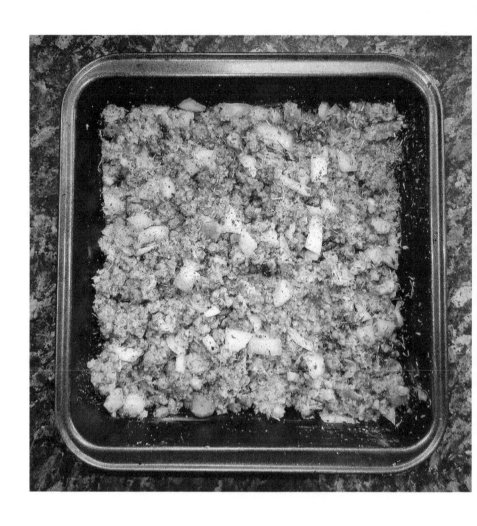

Greek Egg Muffins

Preparation Time: 10 minutes | Cooking Time: 20 minutes | Servings: 12

Ingredients:

6 eggs

1/2 cup feta cheese, crumbled

3 grape tomatoes, chopped

4 sun-dried tomatoes, chopped

2 tsp olive oil

Pepper

Salt

Directions:

In a bowl, whisk eggs with pepper and salt.

Add remaining ingredients and stir everything well.

Pour egg mixture into the 12 silicone muffin molds.

Place the dehydrating tray in a multi-level air fryer basket and place the basket in the Pressure Pot.

Place 6 muffin molds on a dehydrating tray.

Seal pot with air fryer lid and select bake mode then set the temperature to 380 F and timer for 20 minutes.

Bake remaining muffins using the same method.

Serve and enjoy.

Nutrition:

Calories 62, Fat 4.4g, Carbohydrates 2.1g, Sugar 1.2g, Protein 4g, Cholesterol 87mg.

Blueberry Muffins

Preparation Time: 10 minutes | Cooking Time: 20 minutes | Servings: 12

Ingredients:

2 eggs

16 oz cream cheese

1/4 cup blueberries

1/2 tsp vanilla

1/2 cup Swerve

Directions:

Add cream cheese into the mixing bowl and beat until smooth.

Add vanilla, eggs, and sweetener and beat until well combined.

Add blueberries and fold well.

Spoon batter into the 12 silicone muffin molds.

Place the dehydrating tray in a multi-level air fryer basket and place the basket in the Pressure Pot.

Place 6 muffin molds on a dehydrating tray.

Seal pot with air fryer lid and select bake mode then set the temperature to 350° F and timer for 20 minutes.

Bake remaining muffins using the same method.

Serve and enjoy.

Nutrition:

Calories 145, Fat 13.9g, Carbohydrates 1.6g, Sugar 0.5g, Protein 3.8g, Cholesterol 69 mg.

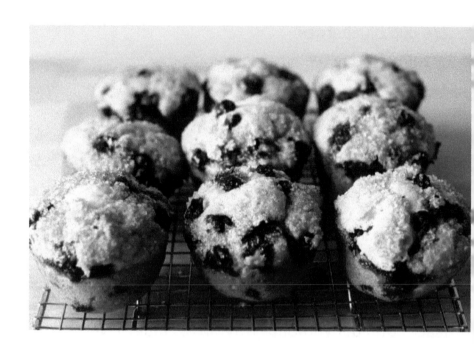

Easy Tarragon Chicken

Preparation Time: 10 minutes | Cooking Time: 12 minutes | Servings: 2

Ingredients:

2 chicken breasts, skinless and boneless

2 tbsp dried tarragon

1 tbsp butter, melted

1/4 tsp garlic powder

Pepper

Salt

Directions:

Brush chicken with melted butter and rub with tarragon, garlic powder, pepper, and salt.

Place the dehydrating tray in a multi-level air fryer basket and place the basket in the Pressure Pot.

Place chicken breasts on a dehydrating tray.

Seal pot with air fryer lid and select air fry mode then set the temperature to 390° F and timer for 12 minutes.

Turn chicken halfway through.

Serve and enjoy.

Nutrition:

Calories 335, Fat 16.7g, Carbohydrates 1.2g, Sugar 0.1g, Protein 42.8g, Cholesterol 145 mg.

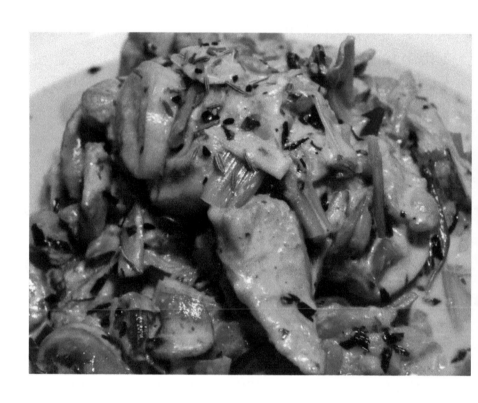

Breaded Turkey Breast

Preparation Time: 10 minutes | Cooking Time: 15 minutes | Servings: 2

Ingredients:

1 turkey breast, skinless and boneless

1/4 tsp cayenne

1/4 tsp garlic powder

1/2 cup breadcrumbs

3 tbsp butter, melted

Pepper

Salt

Directions:

In a shallow dish, mix breadcrumbs, cayenne, garlic powder, pepper, and salt.

Brush turkey breast with butter and coat with breadcrumbs.

Place the dehydrating tray in a multi-level air fryer basket and place basket in the Pressure Pot.

Place turkey breast on dehydrating tray.

Seal pot with air fryer lid and select air fry mode then set the temperature to 390° F and timer for 15 minutes.

Serve and enjoy.

Nutrition:

Calories 11,90, Fat 33.8g, Carbohydrates 58g, Sugar 33.6g, Protein 158.4g, Cholesterol 435mg.

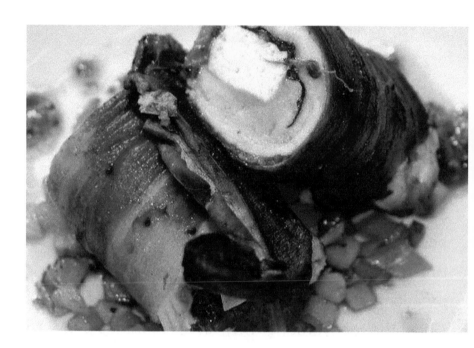

Turkey Patties

Preparation Time: 10 minutes | Cooking Time: 25 minutes | Servings: 8

Ingredients:

1 egg, lightly beaten

2 tbsp lemon juice

2 tbsp cilantro, chopped

1 lb ground turkey

1/3 cup breadcrumbs

1/2 tsp garlic, minced

Pepper

Salt

Directions:

Add all ingredients into the mixing bowl and mix until well combined.

Place the dehydrating tray in a multi-level air fryer basket and place basket in the Pressure Pot.

Make small patties from the meat mixture and place them on a dehydrating tray.

Seal pot with air fryer lid and select bake mode then set the temperature to 380° F and timer for 25 minutes. Turn halfway through.

Serve and enjoy.

Nutrition:

Calories 138, Fat 7g, Carbohydrates 3.4g, Sugar 0.4g, Protein 16.9g, Cholesterol 78mg.

Italian Chicken Breast

Preparation Time: 10 minutes | Cooking Time: 15 minutes | Servings: 1

Ingredients:

1 chicken breast, skinless and boneless

1 tbsp Italian seasoning

1 tbsp olive oil

1 tsp garlic, minced

Pepper

Salt

Directions:

Coat chicken with oil and rub with Italian seasoning, garlic, pepper, and salt.

Place the dehydrating tray in a multi-level air fryer basket and place basket in the Pressure Pot.

Place chicken on the dehydrating tray.

Seal pot with air fryer lid and select air fry mode then set the temperature to 350° F and timer for 15 minutes.

Turn chicken halfway through.

Serve and enjoy.

Nutrition:

Calories 295, Fat 21g, Carbohydrates 2.5g, Sugar 1.3g, Protein 24g, Cholesterol 82mg.

Zucchini Patties

Preparation Time: 10 minutes | Cooking Time: 30 minutes | Servings: 6

Ingredients:

1 egg, lightly beaten

1/2 cup breadcrumbs

2 tbsp onion, minced

1 cup zucchini, shredded

1/4 cup parmesan cheese, grated

1/2 tbsp mayonnaise

Pepper

Salt

Directions:

Add all ingredients into the bowl and mix until well combined.

Place the dehydrating tray in a multi-level air fryer basket and place basket in the Pressure Pot.

Make small patties from the zucchini mixture and place them on a dehydrating tray.

Seal pot with air fryer lid and select bake mode then set the temperature to 380° F and timer for 25 minutes.

Turn patties halfway through.

Serve and enjoy.

Nutrition:

Calories 67, Fat 2.5g, Carbohydrates 7.9g, Sugar 1.2g, Protein 3.6g, Cholesterol 30mg.

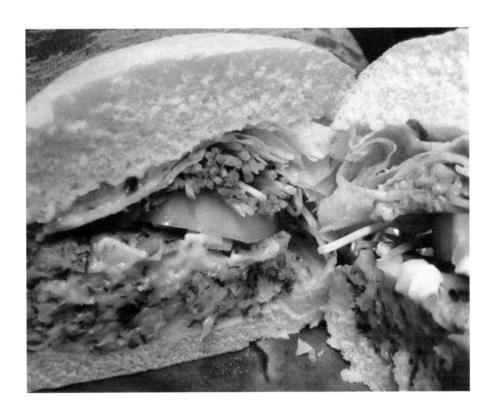

Spinach and Eggs

Preparation time: 25 minutes | Cooking Time: 30 minutes | Servings: 4

Ingredients:

3 cups baby spinach

12 eggs; whisked

1 tbsp. Olive oil

½ tsp. Smoked paprika

Salt and black pepper to taste.

Directions:

Take a bowl and mix all the ingredients except the oil and whisk them well.

Heat your air fryer at 360°F, add the oil, heat it, add the eggs and spinach mix, cover, cook for 20 minutes.

Divide between plates and serve

Nutrition:

Calories 220, Fat 11g, Fiber 3g, Carbs 4g, Protein 6g.

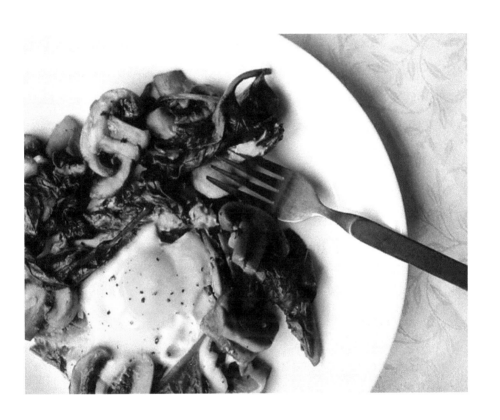

Bell pepper eggs

Preparation time: 25 minutes | Cooking Time: 30 minutes | Servings: 4

Ingredients:

4 medium green bell peppers

¼ medium onion; peeled and chopped

3 oz. Cooked ham; chopped

8 large eggs.

1 cup mild cheddar cheese

Directions:

Cut the tops off each bell pepper. Remove the seeds and the white membranes with a small knife.

Place ham and onion into each pepper

Crack 2 eggs into each pepper. Top with ¼ cup cheese per pepper.

Place into the air fryer basket

Adjust the temperature to 390° F and set the timer for 15 minutes.

When fully cooked, peppers will be tender and eggs will be firm. Serve immediately.

Nutrition:

Calories 314, Protein 24.9g, Fiber 1.7g, Fat 18.6g, Carbs 6.3g.

Cajun Cheese Zucchini

Preparation Time: 10 minutes | Cooking Time: 1 minute | Servings: 4

Ingredients:

4 zucchinis, sliced

1/4 cup parmesan cheese, grated

1/2 cup water

1 tbsp butter

1 tsp garlic powder

1/2 tsp paprika

2 tbsp Cajun seasoning

Directions:

Add all ingredients except cheese into the inner pot of Pressure Pot duo crisp and stir well.

Seal the pot with a pressure-cooking lid and cook on high for 1 minute.

Once done, release pressure using a quick release. Remove lid.

Top with parmesan cheese and serve.

Nutrition:

Calories 80, Fat 4.6g, Carbohydrates 7.4g, Sugar 3.6g, Protein 4.6g, Cholesterol 12mg.

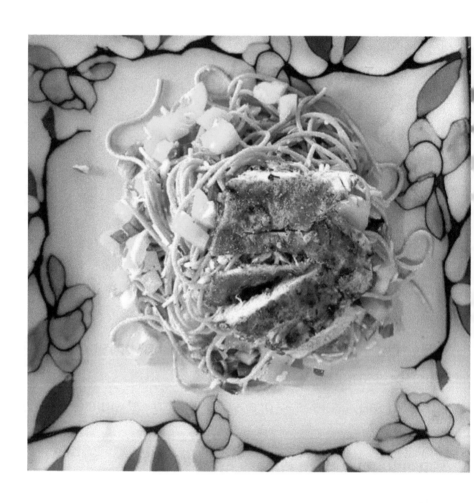

100

Spinach Feta Muffins

Preparation Time: 10 minutes | Cooking Time: 20 minutes | Servings: 6

Ingredients:

3 eggs

1/2 tsp olive oil

1/2 tsp dried oregano

1/2 tsp dried basil

1 tbsp olives, diced

1/4 cup sun-dried tomatoes, diced

2 tbsp spinach, cooked

1/4 cup egg whites

1 tbsp feta cheese, crumbled

Pepper

Salt

Directions:

In a bowl, whisk eggs, oil, and egg whites until well combined.

Add remaining ingredients and stir well.

Pour egg mixture into the silicone muffin molds and place it in the air fryer basket. place basket in the pot.

Seal the pot with an air fryer lid and select bake mode and cook at 350° F for 20 minutes.

Serve and enjoy.

Nutrition:

Calories 55, Fat 3g, Carbohydrates 1.6g, Sugar 0.3g, Protein 4g, Cholesterol 83mg.

Pesto Cheese Chicken

Preparation Time: 10 minutes | Cooking Time: 35 minutes | Servings: 4

Ingredients:

4 chicken breasts, skinless, boneless, and cut in half

1 cup mozzarella cheese, shredded

2 large tomatoes, sliced

1/2 cup basil pesto

Pepper

Salt

Directions:

Line Pressure Pot air fryer basket with aluminum foil and spray with cooking spray.

In a bowl, mix pesto and chicken until coated.

Place chicken in air fryer basket and place basket in the pot.

Seal the pot with an air fryer lid and select bake mode and cook at 400° F for 35 minutes.

Remove chicken from pot and top with cheese and tomatoes.

Serve and enjoy.

Nutrition:

Calories 314, Fat 11g, Carbohydrates 4g, Sugar 2g, Protein 45g, Cholesterol 134mg.

Meatballs

Preparation Time: 10 minutes | Cooking Time: 25 minutes | Servings: 6

Ingredients:

2 lbs ground beef

2 tbsp parsley, chopped

2 tbsp green onion, chopped

1/4 cup bell pepper, roasted and chopped

1/4 cup olives, chopped

1/4 tsp onion powder

1/2 tsp garlic powder

1/4 cup feta cheese, crumbled

1/4 cup sun-dried tomatoes, chopped

1/2 tsp black pepper

1/2 tsp salt

Directions:

Line Pressure Pot air fryer basket with parchment paper or foil.

Add all ingredients into the mixing bowl and mix until combined.

Make small meatballs from the mixture and place them into the air fryer basket. Place basket in the pot.

Seal the pot with an air fryer lid and select bake mode and cook at 400 ° F for 25 minutes.

Serve and enjoy.

Nutrition:

Calories 315, Fat 11g, Carbohydrates 3g, Sugar 0.7g, Protein 46g, Cholesterol 140mg.

Italian Tomato Frittata

Preparation Time: 10 minutes | Cooking Time: 15 minutes | Servings: 4

Ingredients:

6 eggs

1 cup fresh spinach, chopped

1 tsp Italian seasoning

2 tsp heavy cream

1/4 tsp garlic powder

1/4 tsp dried basil

2 bacon slices, cooked and chopped

1/4 cup cherry tomato, halved

1/4 tsp pepper

1/4 tsp salt

Directions:

In a bowl, whisk eggs with Italian seasoning, garlic powder, basil, heavy cream, pepper, and salt.

Spray a 7-inch baking dish with cooking spray.

Add tomato, spinach, and bacon into the prepared baking dish.

Pour egg mixture over tomato spinach mixture. Cover dish with foil.

Pour 1 1/2 cups of water into the Pressure Pot and place the steamer rack in the pot.

Place baking dish on top of the steamer rack.

Seal the pot with a pressure-cooking lid and cook on high for 15 minutes.

Once done, release pressure using a quick release. Remove lid.

Slice and serve.

Nutrition:

Calories 163, Fat 12g, Carbohydrates 2g, Sugar 1.1g, Protein 12g, Cholesterol 260mg.

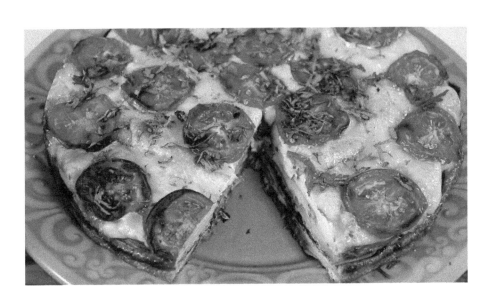

Breakfast Casserole

Preparation Time: 10 minutes | Cooking Time: 30 minutes | Servings: 4

Ingredients:

15 oz breakfast sausage

2 cups of water

1/4 tsp garlic powder

1/2 cup coconut milk

8 eggs, lightly beaten

1 1/2 cups cheddar cheese, shredded

1 onion, diced

1 bell pepper, diced

Pepper

Salt

Directions:

Spray a 7-inch baking dish with cooking spray and set aside.

Add sausage into the inner pot of Pressure Pot and cook on sauté mode until sausage browned.

Add onion and pepper and cook for 2-3 minutes.

Transfer sausage mixture into the prepared baking dish.

Sprinkle cheese on top of sausage.

In a bowl, whisk eggs and milk and pour over sausage mixture. Cover dish with foil.

Pour two cups of water into the Pressure Pot then place the steamer rack in the pot.

Place baking dish on top of the steamer rack.

Seal the pot with a pressure-cooking lid and cook on high for 25 minutes.

Once done, release pressure using a quick release. Remove lid.

Serve and enjoy.

Nutrition:

Calories 424, Fat 32g, Carbohydrates 8g, Sugar 4g, Protein 25g, Cholesterol 458mg.